The Other End
of the Stethoscope

The Other End
of the Stethoscope

33 Insights for Excellent Patient Care

Marcus Engel

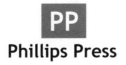

Phillips Press

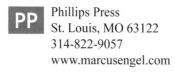 Phillips Press
St. Louis, MO 63122
314-822-9057
www.marcusengel.com

Printed in the United States of America
ISBN: 0-9720000-1-1

ACKNOWLEDGEMENTS

Thanks to any and all medical professionals, both named and unnamed, for giving me part of yourself as I recovered. Even those with whom interactions were not so positive, I am forever in your debt for simply taking care of me when I could not take care of myself.

To my family and friends for helping support me through the darkest times I'll ever know. Some of you took on the care giving responsibilities that are usually only performed by someone with an R.N. or M.D. after their name. Still, you performed your duties with the two things which make up the consummate professional: love and compassion.

To Marvelyne Adams for impeccable editing, beautiful friendship, being my best friend and putting unspoken things into words.

To Jennifer Weaver (www.weaverdesign.net) for turning the words of this manuscript into a visual art.

To all who have read my words or been impacted by my keynotes – your support is what allows me to do what I do.

And, to you, the reader, for taking the time to attempt to better your care by reading my work. You have a special place in my heart for simply doing what you do. Thank you.

TABLE OF CONTENTS

CHAPTER 1

Laying the Groundwork

Scripts of plays are literary fast food. Let's face it: we're American, we like efficiency, we like things "our way, right away," as the Burger King commercial says. I'm no different. You probably aren't, either.

So, I'd like to set this book up as if it were a screenplay. This way, characters don't have to be developed. Right up front, you're told the character's age, sex, personality, and their role in the story; everything you'll need to know. I'll give you all the necessary background info, too. Why? Because scripts for plays take the guesswork out of literature. You don't have to wait for the main character to pick up his cell phone, press a few buttons and talk to his web site manager to figure out that the story takes place in the late 20th or early 21st century. You don't have to get six paragraphs into the story to understand the characters are technologically savvy, white collar computer gurus.

So, here's the rundown on this "play" that stars your old pal, Marcus… and, what's better, you get to be one of the actors. Whether you decide to be a fly on the wall, or put yourself into the shoes of one of the medical professionals, you're part of this story. So, let's get started!

The time: mid-autumn, 1993

The location: Mainly in the hallowed halls of Barnes Hospital, a gigantic fortress smack dab in the heart of St. Louis, Missouri

The main character: Marcus Engel / aka The Patient (that's me, by the way), an 18 year old college freshman. Newly blind, battling through extreme, extreme facial trauma and a variety of other disfiguring and life-threatening injuries; all of which were caused by a drunk driver's irresponsible choice to get behind the wheel. Marcus is angry, frustrated, in horrible pain, and vulnerable – completely vulnerable. He relies on you, his family and other medical personnel for every aspect of his care. He has no choice – he's simply too hurt for any other options.

Supporting cast: Doctors, nurses, therapists, housekeeping staff, radiologists, pretty much anyone who deals with patients like the messed up teenager residing in the ICU and on the plastic surgery floor.

Specifically, there are several health care pros that you'll meet:

Dr. Tim Jones, a plastic surgeon who is either Marcus' best friend, or worst enemy, depending on Marcus' emotion du jour.

Dr. Dennis Fuller, a speech pathologist who gives Marcus the ability to talk after a month of silence. A bear of a man with a booming voice, Fuller never treats Marcus with anything but respect and as the young "dude" that he is.

Dr. Don Gay, a super specialist dentist who can create the ability to eat, even for someone with a mouth as screwed up as Engel's.

Dr. Gene Deune, a plastic surgery resident. (I'll just state right up front that I remember very little about this doctor, so if I have to take a bit of liberty with telling about him, forgive me.)

Dr. Gayle Neely, an ear, nose and throat surgeon with a specialty in ear injuries.

Barb Dewalle, hands down, the best nurse Engel has ever had.

Elaine Slater, Marcus' aunt. Elaine also happens to be a veteran nurse who states, right up front, that her nephew has the worst injuries she's ever witnessed over 25 years of nursing.

Rick, Marcus' only male nurse. Rick treated Marcus not like a patient, but like a guy...a young, single, college guy.

Betty, another great nurse who took an interest in Marcus as a person, not as a patient.

Jennifer, a young woman studying to be a paramedic. Jennifer is the first medical personnel with whom Marcus interacts after being admitted to the hospital.

Overview: Marcus Engel (that's still me) is an 18 year old college freshman at Southwest Missouri State University. He's enjoying his first year of college and the first taste of independence. A typical college freshman; a big guy, over six feet tall, 250 pounds supported on a large frame with wide shoulders which were great when he was playing high school football, but not so great when he wants to buy a suit.

Marcus is moderately good looking, nothing that'd be on the cover of *GQ*, but nothing that causes the opposite sex to turn and run. He's from a small town in mid-Missouri, but left that limited environment behind when he started college.

Marcus has the usual college freshman major: undecided. He's thoughtful, kind, not hasty to make big decisions. Engel doesn't feel he's been exposed to enough of life to declare a major. *Major? No way, not yet!* In the words of Alfred E. Neuman: *What? Me worry?*

Marcus parties with his newfound college friends, but is pretty responsible for being so young. He doesn't skip classes, even if it's been a late night of partying. His grades show his commitment to academics, but don't get the idea that he's the type to live with his nose in a book – at least, not a textbook.

Marcus is a huge music fan, mainly focusing his interest on classic rock from the 60s and 70s. During the weeks he's in Barnes Hospital, music becomes one of Engel's biggest supports. He wholeheartedly believes in Bruce Springsteen's lyric: *We learned more from a three minute record than we ever learned in school.*

Now, let's take a look around his college dorm room; it'll give you a better idea of what sort of person this Marcus guy is (don't worry, he's not here and gives you permission to look around all you want). His dorm room is on the 8th floor of the New Residence Hall at the north end of the

Southwest Missouri State campus. It looks down on Cherry Street which is lined with fraternity and sorority houses, fast food joints and liquor stores. Ah, college convenience!

Most every square inch of wall space on Engel's side of the room is covered with rock posters. A giant black and white head-shot of Bob Dylan peers down at you from high on the west wall. As you glance around, you'll see a monochromatic poster of John Lennon's grave, a Grateful Dead drawing depicting two skeletons sitting on a hill overlooking the San Francisco Bay and, on the backside of his door hangs a full-length black and white of Marilyn Monroe. A tower of CDs rest on top of his desk filled with artists like the Doors, Pearl Jam, Meatloaf, Lynyrd Skynyrd and U2.

A collection of literary works sit on the bookcase; everything from paperbacks of Keats and Dylan Thomas poetry to a gigantic hardcover picture book of Led Zeppelin photos. Under his bed you'll find a few empty beer bottles, an American Eagle backpack, a broom handle he uses for exercises and a spiral notebook from College Algebra; a class Marcus detests and which is taught by what is quite possibly the ugliest woman on earth.

On the corkboard above his desk, there are two photographs, each showing four young men wearing royal blue graduation gowns and mortarboards. These shots were taken in mid-May, just five months before. It was graduation day for Montgomery Co. R-2 High School, Marcus' alma mater. Left to right they are David, Marcus, Jeff and Rodney. These four guys were best of friends through their senior year, all bound for college and something bigger than small town America could offer.

On the top shelf of Engel's bookcase, there are a couple of hairbrushes, sort of useless since his medium brown hair is short enough that it doesn't need much styling. Across the room on the closet, there is a collage of cutouts from magazines. The scraps of paper contain everything from beer advertisements to quotes from poets, pictures of sports cars to athletes and rock stars. Hung over the right hand door of his closet is a Nerf basketball hoop which takes up a significant portion of Engel's time when he should be studying.

The most noticeable thing about this room is that, even with all these pieces that reflect his life, Engel is no where to be seen… and he's never coming back.

Earlier in the week, the cordless phone on his desk rang. The caller, Marcus' buddy, Tom, had an offer that couldn't be turned down: free tickets to the Saturday night hockey match-up between the St. Louis Blues and the Ottawa Senators. Free tickets, Marcus thought, were worth a three hour drive.

It's now Sunday, late morning, and Marcus has been gone a little less than 48 hours. His roommates have no reason to think they won't see him later in the day… or, at least they might be thinking this if they weren't passed out until the early afternoon.

200 miles away, Marcus is clinging to life in a hospital bed, naked except for a cotton sheet covering his mid-section. He does not look like the same attractive young guy that left the dorm two days before. Not at all. In fact, he doesn't even really look human. He still has the arms, legs and torso of a human, but his head… well, it looks like something out of a horror movie. His legs hang in traction above the bed, metal pins piercing his skin at half a dozen

points between his knees and ankles. A tracheostomy has been performed, a trach tube now juts from his throat and an O2 tank hisses nearby with a ghastly sound that reflects just how fragile Marcus' life now is. His body is black and blue, almost head to foot. Red, angry and bleeding scrapes cover his arms, sides and rear. Three-inch wide metal trays are taped over each of his eyes and, below the protection of the flimsy metal, rest two eyes that will never see again. How did Marcus go from that all-American kid to this shell of a human being? Let's step back in time to 12 hours before.

Marcus, Tom and two other friends were headed home after the hockey game. Riding in Tom's Toyota, Marcus took up the shotgun position while Tom drove. The other two teens, Kim and Vince, rode in the backseat. Just south of the hockey arena, and just as Marcus glanced to his right, the foursome saw headlights hurtling toward them. A split second later, the other car ploughed into the passenger side of Tom's Toyota, flipping it several times through the air. All four friends landed outside the car, screaming in pain. Tom and Marcus were a mere four feet apart, but Kim and Vince were crowded onto a grass embankment off to the side of the intersection. The driver of the other car was drunk... not just a little drunk, but completely hammered, stumbling kind of drunk. He refused to take a blood alcohol test. Four hours after the crash a warrant was issued and he was forced to submit to the test. His blood alcohol level showed nearly twice the legal limits of intoxication... and, don't forget, that's after being given four hours to sober up.

At the site of the crash, Marcus is blind. His face is a tangled mess of broken bones, enucleated eyes, cuts and scratches all across his body. His head has swollen to a grotesque size and the paramedics don't know if he'll survive the ambulance ride to the hospital. Simply put, he is one messed up kid. This, my friends, is where we now find ourselves... I, Marcus, the patient, and you, the health care worker, or if you prefer, the fly on the wall.

CHAPTER 2

Two Little Words

I keep hearing sounds; a siren, the clamor of EMS workers, the click of a stretcher as the wheels fall into place. Breaking glass, a woman screaming, the CB radio squawking in the ambulance. I can't put these sounds in order.

I can't listen to them.

I can't pay attention to them.

They just happen.

And they keep happening.

A woman shouts my name and orders me to lay still, the 'whoosh' of automatic doors.

The taste of blood.

A warm blanket.

Pebbles of concrete under my hand.

And pain.

Christ Jesus the pain.

I was blind – immediately, totally, permanently; though no one would say for sure until the surgeons had time to do some exploratory surgery. But, I knew. Deep down, I knew.

Now, here in the emergency room, white hot pain and utter confusion were my guides on the road to hell. Hands ravaged me. Hands everywhere. Cutting off my clothes, re-positioning my body, grabbing my arms and shoving needles into my flesh.

Gallons of morphine were pushed into an I.V., It doesn't stop the pain, but it DOES get me so messed up on narcotics that I don't pay as much attention. The ability to think is completely shot. Memories don't hang around for more than a few seconds – then they're gone.

Exhaustion finally takes over and I fall into uncomfortable sleep. Even when I'm asleep, I hurt. God, the pain!

I awake with a mental crash landing. As soon as I grasp "this"; this horror, this blackness, this rape of every square inch of my body, I'm bludgeoned into seeing white flashes of light. Not truly visual images, but the mental flashbulbs that explode with sudden pain. And they never stop. Paparazzi flashbulb explosions of pain. One after another. Pain is all I know. I surrender to it.

"Marcus? Can you hear me?" asks a female voice.

I dipped my chin. A searing jolt of pain slices my head back into place. I gasp with the pain.

The owner of the voice slips her fingers into my right hand. With her other hand, she lightly traces two fingers up my forearm.

"You're in Barnes Hospital. You were in a car accident," comes the soft voice again, "Just rest now."

I obey. Back into sleep, back to the haunted terrors of hallucination.

Maybe minutes, maybe hours later, I slam back into consciousness. I find the familiar hand from before.

Everything below the neck aches with a dull pain, and everything above burns like dipping my head into a blast furnace. Fear and hurt take over. My breathing kick starts to the rate of a sprinter.

Again, those same questions come from the girl. "Marcus? Can you hear me?"

I'll be damned if I nod again and topple that boulder of pain. Instead, I squeeze the hand. She seems to understand. "Marcus, my name is Jennifer. You're in Barnes Hospital. You were in a car accident," Without thinking, I squeeze the hand again, just to show her I'm getting it.

She pauses. She gives my hand a soft squeeze. Then, the most comforting words of all, "I'm here."

I'm here. I don't even know where "here" is, other than some anonymous name like "Barnes Hospital." But I know I'm not alone. I'm hurt, I'm helpless and I'm scared. I cannot be alone. I cannot be alone. And she's here. This Jennifer girl with her soft hand and quiet voice. She's here.

Jennifer didn't say her title, didn't give her background nor her credentials; just bare bones information. Nothing else was necessary; and she knew it. All I needed to know was that in this world of black – this ocean of pain, I was not alone.

"I'm here." Those two little words are a verbal embrace, a warm, safe place of protection for your patient. When a patient is under your care, they've relinquished all independence, all pride and all their needs to you. Those words, "I'm

here," give an anchor of security and reassurance. No one wants to be alone, especially in an unfamiliar place and with strange things happening. No one wants to be in a hospital, out of their usual element of safety and familiarity. Throw in the pain and fear of whatever their ailment entails and sometimes reassurance is what your patient needs most.

"I'm here" also secures your role as the caregiver. Let's just face it: the patient/caregiver relationship is really that of a child and parent. While the caregiver is on duty, they become the parent. The patient longs for the comfort that all children desire: that their parent is nearby and watching over them.

Those two simple little words often offer more hope and security than anything else you can say or do. As you leave one patient to attend another, use those two little words to reassure your patient that he/she is safe, secure and that all is well. Try it. You'll see their comfort level raise and raise.

CHAPTER 3

Blunt and Focused

"Marc? It's Elaine," says a quiet voice from my right. "Can you hear me?" the voice persists. *Elaine? My Aunt Elaine? The nurse? What's she doing here?* She lives in Chicago, but I'm sure this voice is really her; not a hallucination.

Dude! I must be seriously messed up if Elaine is here, I think, apprehension washing over me.

"Don't try to talk," she said quickly. "You've got a tracheotomy tube in your throat and you can't speak right now." *Well, how can I communicate if I can't talk?*

"Do you think you can write if I give you a pen and some paper?" she asks.

Yes, YES! Of course I can. Give it to me now!

Elaine's voice and words are even, giving no hint of how appalling my appearance is. In a professional manner, which could only come from half a lifetime in the health care field, Elaine swallows her emotions and presses on.

Then, she hands me what will be my means of communication for the next month: a tablet and pencil. The IV needle in the back of my right hand aches as I roll the pencil between my fingers. God, even my fingertips ache.

"Okay, Marc, see if you can write your name."

Slowly, cautiously, I begin to print. I can almost see her biting her lower lip in anticipation. Feeling her eyes on every movement, I try to write legibly.

After finishing my name, I lay the pencil to the side.

"Okay, very good!" Elaine approves.

Pleased I can perform that simple task, she moves onto test number two. "Now, Marc, do you know where you are?" she asks, her voice quiet, but strong. The question is strangely intense.

I don't know it, but she is making a quick clinical assessment of my cognitive functions: Do I recognize who she is? Do I understand her questions? Can I follow commands?

I scan my memory banks for my location. Finally, I latch onto the last place I remember.

"Barnes Hospital?" I wrote with an unsteady hand.

"Yes!" Elaine says clearly encouraged… and maybe a little surprised.

"Now, Marc, do you know why you're in the hospital?"

"Car accident?"

Elaine breathes a long sigh of relief. "Yes!" she says, solidly. What are obvious responses to me are critical, diagnostic pieces of information to her.

"How?" I write, praying she'll understand I wanted details of the crash.

Elaine begins to tell me the details and my mind begins to drift back to that night when a new thought slaps me into focus.

Friends! Terror grabs my throat and begins to squeeze. I'm nearly frantic! I don't even want to think about the possibility, but how can I keep from it?

A single word explodes like a grenade... dead! *They can't be dead! Can they? What if someone really is dead?*

Forcing deep breaths through the trach, I order myself to take control. I still hold the pencil, but I've lost the desire to write... yet I have to. Finally, bracing myself for the answer, I write the question. "How are my friends?"

"Tom is here in Barnes, too. He has some broken bones in his neck and will be in a halo for a long time. Kim has some whiplash and she's wearing a collar, but she's not seriously hurt. Vince is a little beaten up, but he's okay."

The information is bare bones. Elaine knows how shredded one's mind becomes while on morphine. I'm no different. I ask the question again, hoping and praying that I heard everything right. Her answers come back the same as before.

You may, at some point, have to fill your patient in on aspects of life they do not know. The news you give may not be good. The only, ONLY way to give that information is as blunt and focused as possible. Use words that are easy to understand. Do not try to soften any blows. Do not think you'll remove the tragedy by using flowery language. Especially when heavy narcotics are involved, be sure to shorten everything you say. The shorter the response the better. Make short statements and answer questions using an economy of words. You may hold the keys of information, but you can only feed it at the rate the patient can digest it.

CHAPTER 4

Meathooks

"**M**an, Marcus, you've got some big hands! You could hang a side of beef from these meathooks!" a nurse says, smiling, sliding an IV needle into the back of my right hand. "I'm used to working on little old ladies who have these tiny little veins. You've got these big, thick veins the size of fire hoses! You make my job easy!"

I'm still too hurt to smile, but I do smirk a bit on the inside. I like this nurse. She's not treating me like a fragile invalid, but like the tough, football playing guy I'd been just days before. And that idea of meathooks for hands? Yeah, that's a compliment. I like her.

The ripping sound of tape fills my ears. Her hand gently lifts mine and I feel a piece of tape spread over the IV catheter. "There ya go, Marcus! I'm going to give your meathooks back to you now. Hit your nurse call button if you need anything, okay?" I nod and wish she would stay with me. She cannot, but she does appear every so often to check in on me.

And every time, she says, "Hey, Meathooks! How are ya?" I cannot respond, other than with some hand signals. I lift one hand and wave it side to side, trying to make a sign that shows I'm hearing her, but not doing so well. She understands. "I'll give you some pain killer," she says, and lightly grasps my fingers to get a better view of my IV. "I'm telling ya, Meathooks, you have the biggest hands I've seen in a long time!" Her tone is complimentary. I grin inside. I'm doing better now. She recognizes that I'm young, that I was strong before this horrible crash, and she's giving me some reason to believe I'm still a stud, if I ever was one in the first place!

"Meathooks." This nickname indicated strength, toughness and power — something I'd been before, but not how I felt post-crash. Still, my former self would have loved the nickname had it been given in a locker room, Now, I just loved it because it showed this nurse had a special place for her young patient with big hands.

Do I remember her name? No. But, do I remember how she cared for me? You bet! Did she do anything different than the other nurses? Not necessarily, but she certainly gave me an identity that allowed me to retain a sense of my previous self. That was worth more than the most gentle of care.

Through the rest of my hospitalization, I'd receive nicknames like "Dude," "Wild Man," "Buddy Bud" and a variety of others. After a decade, many of my caregivers have slipped from memory, but those who dubbed me with a nickname will never be forgotten. With such a great number of specialists always examining me, at first, it was difficult to differentiate them. Those who stuck me with a title or nickname were easily identifiable.

Remember your childhood nicknames? Usually, nicknames come from one of two types of people: those who love you, or those who hate you. As a patient's caregiver, you should fall into the former. If you have a long term patient, think about coming up with a nickname for that person, preferably one that's exclusive and flattering. If it isn't flattering, feel out the patient's personality before dubbing them with something that might be offensive. With the horrible amounts of facial damage, nicknaming me on strength was good, but any title that drew attention to my ruined looks would not have been accepted. No health care provider could have gotten away with nicknaming me "Handsome" or "Cutie."

Also, nicknaming patients is a way to secure that person's presence in your mind. If you're taking care of half a dozen elderly women during a shift, a nickname might help you remember who has been cared for at what time, what their vitals were and if there was any cause for concern. Try it! The more you work at this, the better you'll become at creating these new handles!

CHAPTER 5

Privacy

Pee. Yup, pee. It's one of the first words children learn. Why? Because we all do it, we all need to do it several times per day, and we all feel better after doing it. So, pee.

From a very young age, we know that there is a right way and a wrong way to pee. The wrong way is in our pants, the bed, anything that might be slightly messy. The toilet! That's where the pee goes!

Take an adult who has been using a toilet for their bodily needs for, oh, say the last 20 years or so. Then, hand them a big plastic jug and tell them to pee in it. Further that pressure by telling them their pee will be tested and measured following nature's call. Then, just to make them feel even more uncomfortable, why not hang around and watch, throwing in little comments like, "Need any help?" Did I forget to mention that urination must also be done while laying flat in a bed? Oh, the pressure!

The 1000 cc plastic pitcher, after only one use, became known by its more accurate name, *The Piss Jug*.

For the first several weeks of silence due to the trach, the number of times "piss jug" was written across a page is immeasurable. Gallons of IV fluid and nothing but clear liquids by mouth added up to one thing: pee. And lots of it!

Even though I needed help to position the piss jug, the nurse was kind enough to give me 30 seconds of solitude.

"I'm going to step into the hall to give you some privacy. Just hit your call light when you're done," she says, stopping for just a moment to witness my slight nod of recognition.

She exits. I pee. The world becomes a better place.

Since potty training, we've learned that going #1 and #2 are to be done in private. Due to circumstances, hospitals don't always allow for that social norm. Maybe the patient can't get out of bed, maybe your patient can't use a traditional toilet, maybe there isn't a bathroom in the room, whatever reason, the standard we've known since we were toddler's flies out the window. A piss jug is de-humanizing, a commode is humiliating and having to use anything but a traditional toilet in a traditional way is the fastest way to have one's spirit broken.

If you can prevent any embarrassment or discomfort for your patients by turning away, leaving the room for half a minute or, if nothing else, providing a sheet or curtain to cover them, do it. This is one of the fastest ways to get this individual "on your side." Depending on the age of your patient, different measures may need to be taken, but offering them some privacy is the very essence of helping them. Your patients will love you for helping them retain some degree of modesty and dignity; even if they're too embarrassed to consciously thank you for it.

CHAPTER 6

Common Ground

I am in a daze. 25 hours of surgery will do that to a person, I suppose. The nurses and orderlies wheel me out of the elevator and down the hall. My parents are here. Mom has been crying. I'm too tired and out of it to do anything but notice the obvious.

"Marc, this is a new place," Dad says. "You were down on the sixth floor, but this is now the 7400 floor." I shrug and lift one finger, just to show his words are sinking in.

There are nurses and people everywhere. There is one in particular who seems to be the leader. "Marc, we're going to step out until they get you settled in," Dad says. "We'll be back in a few minutes." I nod, or at least try to. My head feels like it's three feet wide. The pain is enormous. The nurse, the one who is in charge, speaks to me.

"Okay, we're going to lift you with the sheet under you and help get you off the gurney and into your new bed." I'm too weak to protest or ask questions. I nod again, just to show I understand. A few minutes later, the task is complete. The orderlies exit, the nurse, who I've learned is named Barb, situates pillows and blankets across my body. After a few moments of idle chit chatting with her mute patient, she asks a direct question.

"Where'd ya go to high school?"

"Montgomery county, R-II," I scrawl onto my tablet.

"Where is that?" Barb asks, sounding puzzled.

"Halfway to Columbia," I write. "The friends I was with in the crash go to Lindbergh and Mehlville."

"Oh yeah? I live in south county, and my kids go to Mehlville, too," she says, smiling.

Bingo! Immediate connection! We had, in less than 60 seconds, found common ground.

For those not from our fair city, you may think Barb asked about my high school because I was a teenager. Negative. This question, "Where'd ya go to high school?" seems exclusively a St. Louis thing. And it's not just with those who are in high school. Old men, 50 years past graduation will ask one another this all-important question. It gives an idea of one's socio-economic background, level of intelligence and offers a potential connection with a mutual acquaintance. It was the perfect question for Barb to ask.

Whether it's two businessmen making a connection at a meeting, or a patient and nurse bonding over high school trivia, it is of the utmost in importance. The shortest distance between two individuals is a laugh, but the second shortest distance is something in common. Even if nothing dramatic pops up, the caregiver's questions show interest in the patient as an individual, not just another body to be treated. Questions, connections and common ground are vital tools in assisting your patient to feel like a whole person, and helping them remember you are too.

CHAPTER 7

"What Do You Go By?"

M an, Marcus. I've gotta tell you, you've gotten hurt pretty bad," Barb says. She's already become one of my favorite nurses. "In fact, I'm not sure I've ever seen a patient who has been hurt quite as badly as you," she says.

I'm not 100% sure how to take this, but I decide it's a compliment. After all, I've now lived through a worse trauma than anyone else this veteran nurse has treated.

"Your parents went down to the cafeteria, Marcus, but they'll be back soo..." her voice trails off.

"Do you prefer to be called 'Marc' or 'Marcus'?" She stops and looks directly at me.

"Either one, but my name is spelled with a *C*," I write. I trace three dark lines under the *C* for emphasis.

"Gotcha then, Marc. Anyway, your parents will be back soon. I told them I'd tell you where they went if you woke up before they got back. Can I get you anything, Marc?"

I am anxious to get to know this woman. She is confident but casual, professional and personable. She's not worried about treating me like a fragile little antique or something. And... she actually cares about my name!

One's name is completely tied to their identity. Hollywood celebrities know this and often change their name to something more memorable. Would you associate Henry John Deutschendorf with the majestic Rocky Mountains? Probably not, but you might if his name is John Denver. People typically like their name. If they don't, they find some sort of handle that IS acceptable. If you ask your patient what he/she prefers to be called, you are abiding by an all important rule of care — treating the patient like a person.

Barb's concern over my preference was an important part of making me feel like she recognized me as an individual, and it was also important to me as a teenager. One does not typically call a teen "Mister" anything. Yet, there I was, fighting adult problems in an adult ward in an adult hospital. And I'm still a teenager. By allowing me to retain my status as a young man, Barb was helping to carve out a place in my mind that I was still young, still alive and I still had a lot of growing up to do. I wasn't yet a "Mister" nor was I a "sir." I was just "Marc." That made the biggest difference to me, and it will to your patients, too.

CHAPTER 8

Sacrificing the Messenger

"I'm blind?" I write out, slow and deliberate.

"Yes," comes the ophthalmologist's one word reply. It is sure, it is definite and leaves no escape.

"You can't do anything else? No transplants or exercises? Nothing?" I scrawl. Praying they've overlooked something.

"No, Marcus, there's nothing we can do. And, there's nothing you can do, either. I'm sorry…" his voice trails off. His helplessness sharply contrasts his sure manner of speaking.

This is not happening, I think, fear and anger growing, *I cannot believe this!* Shock gives way to surprise which gives way to frustration. *Some of the best doctors in the world are looking at my eyes and they can't save my sight?*

I grab my pencil. *These incompetent, useless bastards.* I'm ready. Ready to tell them so.

"How can you even look at yourself? I HATE YOU!" I scrawl darkly across the page. Seething with white hot anger, I swear and swear and swear at these fools that call themselves doctors.

Bastards! Fix me, dammit! I scream through a brain full of chemicals.

I can almost see the looks that pass between the physicians and my family. That look that says, "I'm sorry. I'm so sorry." With quiet resignation, the physicians slip away from the bedside. My family moves in and provides the only comfort they can: human touch.

Without waiting for dismissal, the ophthalmologists quietly leave the room.

Does anyone like being sworn at? Does anyone like to be reminded of their failings? Or that they're helpless? Of course not! In the role of a caregiver, you'll be hit with these sorts of insults. How do you handle them? Become calloused? Spit back anger at the patient? Explain how their anger is misplaced and that you are not to blame for their current predicament? No, no and no.

Deep down, every patient knows their ailment does NOT lie at the feet of their caregivers. Does that mean they'll accept it? Nope! Think of it: Your patient is suffering. Maybe heavy painkillers are disrupting their thought processes. They feel unable to control any aspect of life. They'll probably have a hard time dealing with their current infirmity. Wouldn't you? And, who is the nearest person they can take it out on? You. You, the caregiver. You, the bearer of the brunt of the patient's hostility. You, the person who only wants to help, will be cursed at, spat upon, screamed at and told every flaw that you possess, as well as some you don't. And the reason is simple. You're a safe place. Be ready.

Then, begin to think of yourself as the sacrificial lamb. Know that your patient is likely to "kill the messenger." Your patient needs that initial vent session. Don't hold it against them, even if they hold it against you. Don't think every time you step into their quarters you'll be hit with that same degree of anger. Maybe it'll happen, maybe not, but sacrificing your pride by biting your tongue may get the patient to push that venom out of his/her system. The last thing a patient needs is a lecture on their poor behavior. They already know that behavior is deplorable.

Under stressful, painful circumstances, even someone who generally is quiet and demure may turn into a raging jerk. Their insults are misdirected. You know this. They may not be able to comprehend it at this time. Hard as it may be, swallow their ambush with graciousness. Then, erase it from memory as quickly as possible. Easier said than done, but remember part of your service to the patient is allowing that person to retain as much control as possible - even if that control insults you.

CHAPTER 9

No, You Don't Know How They Feel, So Don't Say It!

"**M**arcus, I know what you're going through. I, too, was in a car accident when I was 24. I broke my back and I was in bed for three months. I know what you're going through," the nurse says. Every word that comes from her mouth infuriates me even more. She knows how I feel? Oh really? Because she's a teenage guy? Because she was 24? Because no doctor ever came in and told her she'd never see again? Right. The similarities are just endless. I wanted to hit her.

How many times has someone told you, "I know how you feel"? You're facing some sort of adverse situation and, in a desire to provide some comfort, someone blurts out that idiotic phrase: "I know how you feel!" No, no you don't. Unless you have been in that exact situation, unless you've faced down identical practices, and unless you've lived inside that person's mind with all the socialization and psyche that makes up their personality, no, no you don't know how they feel. So, don't say you do.

Sure, when someone says this, his or her heart is in the right place, but there is no way, absolutely no way, anyone can know exactly how another feels.

In Christopher Reeves' autobiography, he tells a story of a letter he received from a fan, after the horseback riding incident that left him paralyzed from the neck down. The fan claimed she knew what he was going through because she'd had chronic diarrhea her entire life. What? What sort of asinine comment is that?

Now, instead of playing the empathy card, think of a better way to show you sympathize with the patient's situation. Try these on for size:

"There's no way I can know what you're going through, but I want you to know I'm here to help you however I can." Or maybe, "This seems so unbearable for you, and I want you to know that if you need anything at all, just let me know."

By these comments, you're showing the person you recognize them as an individual, with a unique set of emotions and reactions, not just a patient on your case load. Give it a try... or at least don't tell them "I know what you're going through."

CHAPTER 10

Embrace the Oddity

"**M**arcus, I'm Lisa."

Lisa? Lisa who?

"You're in the ICU. Your doctor ordered a nurse to be posted by your bed for the next 24 hours. That's why I'm here. Is there anything you need?"

I grip an imaginary pencil and scrawl some invisible lines in the air. The clipboard and tablet are the only means I have of communicating, and those are no where within my grasp.

"Here ya go," Lisa says, flipping over a fresh sheet of paper.

"What happened?" I write. My hand is unsteady with morphine.

"You had another major surgery. They knew it would be long, but you were in the O.R. for nearly 20 hours."

Twenty hours? A vague memory of the recovery room drifts around my mind, elusive as a trophy salmon to a fisherman.

"Since it was such a big surgery, the doctors wanted someone to keep a close eye on you. So, I'm here! My only job is to watch you tonight, kiddo," Lisa says, a smile creeping to her lips.

"I'm awake now," I write, hoping she'll understand my body has had about all the sleep it can stand.

"No problem, Marc. I'm here if you need anything," Lisa says, settling back into her command post.

"Can you talk to me?" I ask. I need human contact, need to know my caretaker is trustworthy, need to know I am not alone.

"Sure, no problem. I brought this book along tonight to read while you were sleeping. How about I just read it out loud? It's 'Different Seasons' by Stephen King. I'm about halfway through one of the stories, but I can start over if you want."

Stephen King: killer clowns, monsters that live in sewers, rabid dogs, murderous cars with minds of their own. Stephen King stories on morphine is NOT a good idea.

"Can you just talk to me? Morphine makes me hallucinate. It's scary. I don't want to be scared any more."

"Yeah, you're right, Marc. That does sound like a bad idea. So, what do you want to talk about?" Lisa asks, smiling at how our interaction is starting out.

"Tell me about you," I write. Every caregiver is questioned about his/her pedigree and competency.

"Well, I've been a nurse for 10 years, but I only come in when the hospital needs me. I have two little boys at home and I just decided I wanted to watch them grow up instead of working full time," she smiles at the thought of her boys.

I nod. Good, I think, someone who has their priorities straight when it comes to taking care of people.

"Marcus, you said you've been having hallucinations. What are they like?" she asks cautiously, probably feeling like she's stepping onto thin ice.

"They're all really weird. I thought I was in a grocery store, I thought one of my friends was a bear, I thought I was in an ocean. While ago, I saw all these people standing around looking at me. Probably 20 or more. They just kept looking at me," I write. It feels good to tell someone about these things; makes me feel more grounded to reality.

"Do you think they're people from the accident?"

"No, I don't know them. None of them. There's also a dog, a cocker spaniel, I think, and he's running around my feet. The floor is carpet and is really dirty. He's not mean or anything, but I can't touch him."

"Do you have a dog at home? Think that might be your dog you keep seeing?"

"No, it's not mine. I have a beagle, but she's fat and old. The weird thing is that I can't move. I can't touch the dog and I can't walk away from the people."

"Well, you're kinda tied up in this bed now, so that might be why you can't move in your dreams, too," she ventures.

"I don't know. I just don't know…"

This was the only night I spent under Lisa's care. The only night. Yet, our conversations are im-printed in my memory. She didn't have that many duties, mainly just to keep an eye on my vitals and alert the doctors if there was any change. Yet, she is such a part of the hospital memory banks. Why? Because she provided some relief from boredom? Because she gave me some vital information that no one else had bothered to tell me? Because she helped me pass the hours after my body was saturated from sleep? Yes to all of those, but the biggest thing Lisa did was engage me in the manner I needed to talk. She wasn't afraid of the conversation.

Hallucinations? Dogs? Grocery stores? Strangers? So often, people sweep oddities under the rug. Not Lisa. She allowed me to embrace the oddity of the situation, listened, asked questions and tried to help me figure out why I was hallucinating such crazy things.

Don't ever be afraid to talk to your patients about what they want to discuss. In school, we always heard, "There are no such things as stupid questions." Maybe not, but sometimes we are afraid of things we don't know. Even if I was high as a kite while Lisa was at my bedside, she knew that talking about my hallucinations wouldn't make matters worse. Nothing your patient asks will make his/her situation worse. Allow them to talk the way they need - and listen. And engage them. And you'll make their next few hours a little more tolerable.

CHAPTER 11

Smile

"Hey Marcus," the medical tech says, shuffling up to my bed. "It's time for your bath."

His tone isn't unfriendly, but he does sound, well, bored. Granted, I may not be excited about giving a man a bath either, but his enthusiasm level is just at zero. I scrawl, "NO!" onto the tablet.

"You don't want your bath?" he says. Is that hopefulness I hear in his voice? I point at the page where I'd just written my wish. He ignores it. He has a job to do, whether I want it done or not. He fills a pan of water at the sink and sets it down on the bedside table. Never once does he smile, laugh or act the least bit interested. Of course I don't want him acting like the class clown while bathing me, but with his disinterested detachment I feel like a burden. I don't want to be a burden. But I know I am. And his lack of enthusiasm makes me feel even worse.

How often have you walked up to someone that had a huge frown plastered across their mug, stuck out your hand and said, "Hi there! Nice to meet you!" Rarely, if ever, I'll bet.

Now, reverse that situation. Let's say you're walking along and see someone who has a giant grin written across their face. Don't you wonder, "What's she so happy about?" or "What's his secret?"

Smiles are only the movement of a few facial muscles. Yet, that very, very small effort on your part makes you appear more attractive and trustworthy, and even (dare I say?) causes you to feel more happiness yourself. If you're not in a great mood, well, at least try to look like it's not the end of the world! No one wants to be under the care of a disgruntled person.

A simple smile when you walk in the room and a short couple of sentences that explain your role and duties, that's all it takes! And that's all it would have taken for this med tech to be in my good graces. Had he smiled when he said, "Hey, Marcus!" and put just a little enthusiasm in his voice, he would have helped the entire environment.

Of the vast amount of medical personnel who surrounded my bedside during those months, it was the ones who smiled and introduced themselves that I remember most. Those were the folks who got less complaints, more thanks and favorable reports when the follow-up calls came from the hospital.

Try it! It's the quickest way for your patient to get a good first impression of the kind of care he/she will receive while on your watch.

CHAPTER 12

Information - Bit by Bit

"I want to know about my legs," I scrawl on my tablet. Rita, my nurse, looks down at my words. For the previous two weeks, my legs have hung in traction above the bed. Pins penetrate the bones of my left leg, but I don't know how many, where they're placed, anything. I want to know, but if Rita gives me too much information, such as, "You've got 30 pins hanging out, they're all bloody and gross and look like something out of a horror movie," well, I'd be better in my world of blissful ignorance.

"Okay," Rita says slowly, measuring her words.

"Please don't tell me too much too fast," I scrawl, immediately putting her on caution alert.

"Okay, what would you like me to tell you, Marcus?"

"Just answer yes or no. If I want more of an explanation, I'll ask. Cool?"

"Sure, no problem," she says, taking time to be sure my request is met.

"Are there pins in my feet?" I ask.

"No, there are not."

"Where is the lowest pin?"

"The lowest pin is at your ankle," she replied.

"How far up is the next pin?"

"Around four or five inches above your ankle," she says, her voice slowing so she doesn't blurt out the wrong thing.

"Okay. Where is the highest pin?"

"The top pin is through your knee."

"So, all the pins in my legs are between the knee and ankle?"

"Yes," she states, the barest bones of information only given at my chosen rate of ingestion.

"How many pins are there total?"

"The grand total of pins between your knee and ankle is four. That's all."

I exhale deeply. Then once more. It is the breath of someone who holds their breath, waiting for bad news. Then, the bad news turns out not to be so bad.

"Okay, good. Where are each of them?" Now, I'm confident in her abilities to only give the particles of information I desire.

"Your left ankle has a pin, then four inches above the ankle is another. At the exit site where the break occurred is another. Finally, the top pin is at your knee. There are only four, Marcus."

Again, I let out a long breath.

Every day, nurses came in six or seven times per day to do what they termed, "pin care." It meant nothing more than cleaning the exit sites for each pin with peroxide and then daubing each with a topical anti-biotic salve. Doing this so often got me really concerned about what was going on with my legs. Not being able to see anything, and feeling some slight stings as the peroxide was applied really made me wonder just what they were doing down there.

If you've ever had surgery, you may remember the first viewing of the incision post-surgery. Remember being a little scared to remove the dressing, pull off the tape and take a gander at where the surgeon had opened up your body?

Now, imagine being unable to remove the tape yourself. Think of the inability to pull the tape off and being unable to re-attach the dressing if the wound beneath is too frightening.

Your patient may be curious, but they may also want to digest the repairs to their body bit by bit, not having everything heaped on a plate at once and force fed. Asking how they'd like to receive information about their medical condition is always, always a good plan. Starting slow, using specific and measurable terms, stopping immediately if they show revulsion, is always the best way to handle this situation. Remember, if your patient is thirsting for knowledge, do not give them a drink with a fire hose.

CHAPTER 13

Vital Compliments

There is a loud ripping sound as Barb pulls off the blood pressure cuff. I flex my fingers into a quick fist, then release.

"Your blood pressure is 115 over 75, Marcus. That's right where it should be for a young, healthy guy like yourself!" I smile.

"I've gotta get your temp, too," she says. I tilt my head to the left, offering up my right ear. A cold, metal pyramid slides into my ear canal, just enough to feel uncomfortable. A couple of quick beeps emit from the thermometer and Barb gently pulls it away. It's over.

"98.6. That's excellent!" she beams. I smile again.

Freshman year biology taught me what a human's body temperature should be. I feel anything but human. But when Barb tells me my temp and says it's "excellent," then maybe, just maybe I'm still human.

At 18, the only times I'd had my blood pressure taken was during a physical for football, or on one of those big machines at K-Mart that looks more like an arcade game than a medical device. Either way, these numbers over numbers were Greek to me. So, Barb educated me. "115 over 75" and "That's right where it needs to be" gave me the specifics, but also gave me the target. I was in that target range, and she further boosted my esteem by calling me a "young, healthy guy."

Your average patient is probably not all that different from me. I'll wager that the majority of folks have no idea what their blood pressure is, nor where it ranks on the scale. Unless your patient has had extensive medical history or complications, they are probably quite ignorant of where their vitals rank.

The only thing worse than telling your patient something he/she doesn't understand is not telling them anything at all! If a nurse takes vitals and scribbles them on my chart without verbalizing what she found, I feel like something is being hidden. No one likes being kept in the dark, but that's even less acceptable when what's being hidden deals directly with a patient's status as a human being. "It's my body and I deserve to know what it's doing!" I wanted to scream when the vitals weren't given.

Since most patients do not have the medical background to know that 120 over 80 is a perfect blood pressure, it's your job to tell them. Then, reassure your patient with a little compliment.

"Your blood pressure is perfect!" Or, "Your temperature is 98.6. That's right where it should be!"

Now, what other vitals do you deal with? Pee? This is one you may have to dance around, but when emptying a patient's urine bag, tell them the amount. "Mr. Smith, there was about 700 CCs in your urine bag. Your output is good and your urine looks healthy." Kind of gross to compliment the color of someone's pee? Maybe, but consider it prophecy. Your patient will now know that at least one part of his body is healthy! Share the information, compliment their measurements and watch your patient heal!

CHAPTER 14

Confidence:
There's Nothing Like It!

"Marcus! Hey, how ya doing?" the voice thunders from above. Not only is it loud, but this voice is... smiling? Really? Surprised by the brazen entrance, I recoil. I had been awakened out of a sound sleep by this booming voice stretching overhead. I try to focus. I'm still groggy from sleep, but I decide I'm more intrigued than annoyed. The baritone comes from higher than the usual voices around my bed. Whoever this new guy is, he's tall. And something is different... almost interesting! Whoever he is, he has a powerful presence – very powerful.

The voice booms again, "My name is Dennis Fuller and I'm a speech pathologist. I'm going to do a little work with your trach here and see if we can get you talking."

As he introduces himself, he grabs my right hand and shakes it with a crushing grip. Whoever this guy is, he's definitely not going to baby me! I almost smile!

Even with his enormous presence, I'm not the slightest bit concerned this new doc will inflict any more pain. But, what is really intriguing is what he just said. *Talking again?*

After three weeks of silence, I'll be able to talk? I sit, too stunned to move. In the three weeks that have elapsed since the crash, this is about the only good news I've received!

"Okay, Dude," Dennis says, examining some device at the side of the bed. *Dude? Did this guy just call me dude?* "Dude" was what Dennis came to call me on a regular basis. Formality is obviously unnecessary when a physician calls me, "dude."

"Okay, Dude." Dennis repeats, holding the collar around my neck. Dennis clicks a piece into place. "Okay, done!" he says with a magician's flare. *Huh? Done? That only took a few seconds!*

"Since you're breath won't be taking a shortcut through your throat, you'll be able to talk again, okay?"

I scrawl "Okay" in response.

"No way, Dude. You're not getting off that easily!" He mocks anger. "I want you to say 'Okay.' So, take in a deep breath and say the word."

I wait a second or two, draw in a deep breath and utter the first audible sounds in three weeks.

The single biggest reason Dennis could get me to work hard at speech therapy was due to one thing: his confidence, in himself, in the equipment and in me. Had he come into my room and meekly said, "Excuse me, Marcus? I'm your speech pathologist and I need to do some things to your trach, okay?" I'd have given him the boot. But, his self confidence, in turn, made me think failure wasn't an option.

Never be meek to a patient. That person will smell insecurity and fear like a fart in a car. Patients want to know their physicians and caregivers know what they're doing. No better way to show someone that than to treat them as if they aren't lying in a hospital bed. Dennis started our interaction with a handshake. Not some limp-wristed handshake you'd give a senior citizen, but a manly handshake that made me feel like an able bodied possessor of the x & y chromosome! That was the sort of handshake he could give to a fellow doctor, or a WCW wrestler, or practically anyone that was NOT laying in a hospital bed. Yet, he gave it to me, fear and uncertainty be damned! Show confidence in yourself and it will quickly build confidence in your patient, too.

CHAPTER 15

Gifts

The phone by my bed rings. I stretch out an IV tube lined arm and pick the receiver off the cradle. "Low" has to suffice as "hello." The talking trach just went in yesterday. This is my first real test to see if someone can understand me. Whoever is on the other end doesn't have the back-up of me writing responses on the tablet.

Strangely, it's Betty, one of my nurses. "Marc, I'm going to the music store this afternoon. Is there anything I can get you?" I am shocked. Betty is my nurse on duty almost every night. She is not, however, what I think of as a friend. I expect her to take care of me while she's working. I do not expect her to do my shopping for me.

I fumble through a response that sounds like, "No, not really." Betty knows I can't talk and doesn't continue the conversation. "Well, I'll see if I can find something you'll like," She says. The phone clicks. I hang up.

My mind flashes back to the night before. Betty had been on duty. Through my new talking trach, I rasped out, "Led Zeppelin," but it sounded like "led zeflun." I tapped my finger on one of the many tapes lined up by the portable boom box, indicating which tape I wanted her to pick out and pop in the player. She understood. Then, we'd talked a bit while she looked over my collection of music. Our taste was not the same, by any means, but it meant a lot for my caregiver to take an active interest in something I loved.

The next day is the usual routine; meds, bath, doctors, nurses, more doctors, more nurses, physical therapy, speech therapy, pain, anger, more doctors and nurses, same story, different day. I'm thankful when five o'clock hits and the usual tormentors go home.

Betty is back on duty tonight. She pops into my room and brings me a tape. Simon and Garfunkel's **Concert in Central Park**. My dead eyes fill with tears. It is only a $10 tape, but this means the world to me. She has no idea how awful today has been, no idea how I've spent the day being pissed off at every doctor and nurse and therapist who has taken up my time, no idea how many times I've wished I was dead. Yes, it's been just that bad. Now? Now I get this unsolicited gift from the most unlikely of benefactors. I will treasure this. She can't know what this means to me. She just can't. She's never laid in this bed, helpless. She's never wanted to go outside so badly she can almost taste it. She's never seen people bend over backwards to make her life just the tiniest bit brighter. And she can't know how much this makes me love her.

I'd been the biggest ingrate of a patient; pissed off, shouting, swearing, general hatefulness spewing at my caregivers. Why? Were they that bad? No, but I had no one else to take it out on. Ingrate. Ingrate. Ingrate. That's exactly what I am. Not any more. Not to Betty, at least.

Should a caregiver get their patients presents? "Yeah, right," you're thinking. "How can someone afford gifts for a multitude of patients on my salary? My job is to take care of people in the hospital, not to take the place of Santa Claus." True, and no one is asking you to.

What did that call take? Two minutes and ten bucks. Was it necessary? Nope, that's why it meant so much. Trust me about this... your patient will appreciate it in ways you may never know. After that, do you think I ever, ever did anything that would make Betty's job harder? Not even close. Every time she came in, she knew she was going to have a patient that was meek as a lamb. Bribery? Sure! Did it work? Absolutely! Should other caregivers do it? Debatable, but nothing will ever get a patient on "your side" like a little cheap bribe!

CHAPTER 16

Rock the Boat...
for the Right Reasons

It's 3 a.m. I can't sleep. I woke up at 4 a.m., almost 24 hours ago. The only sleep between now and then came thanks to the nurses who guarded my room to let me nap. Still, that hour of rest was a long, long time ago.

I try to fall asleep. Then, I try harder. Nothing works. Counting sheep, meditation, Benadryl, dammit, nothing works. I need sleep. I need it now. I need a sleeping pill, and I need it so badly I can almost taste it. Frustration is busting within me, and in another 30 minutes, if I don't fall asleep, I'm going to be a basket case. Finally, after about a million sheep and enough deep breathing exercises to hyperventilate, I hit the nurse call light. Thankfully, a nurse appears within a couple of minutes.

"I can't sleep!" I grunt at her. She doesn't know how long I've laid here, how I'm at wit's end. How can she? Still, when I ask for a sleeping pill, I don't receive the response I need.

"Marcus, I'll have to call the house doctor. He'll have to look over your charts and be sure there's no drug interaction. If he says it's okay, he'll write a script, but it's going to take at least an hour to get up here. Are you sure you want me to ask him?"

Are you sure you want me to ask him? This question takes the weight off of her and puts it on MY shoulders. It doesn't take a genius to figure out this is a hassle. A gigantic pain in the neck. She has to go through at least a four step process to even get the pill cleared to go into my body. A hassle, yes. Do I really want to bother her? No, of course not — but I need sleep a whole, whole lot more than she needs to have a hassle-free night on the floor.

Sleep. Sleep is required to be healthy. In a hospital, this is doubly important. A person taken out of their own environment, subjected to surgeries and ailments and the stresses of medical issues needs sleep. When it comes to your patient's comfort level, especially concerning sleep, do whatever needs to be done. If the doctor on duty gets upset about being called out to prescribe a sleeping pill, so be it. That patient's healing is your #1 concern. Never, EVER disregard a patient's need due to your desire not to rock the boat. When it is necessary, rock the boat — your patient is depending on it.

CHAPTER 17

Over-Apologize? Never!

"**O**h my God! That burns like hell!" I wail and pound my arms into the bed. I grind my fists into the mattress, bludgeoning them harder and harder. I crunch my jaws together and wince and wait and pray. I will the burning to pass.

It's Hepron. Blood thinner. And it's the time of day I dread.

"This has to be injected into a fatty area, Marcus," the nurse said before this wretched experience began. Dilemma: The most fatty area of me is my belly… and the thought of needles in my gut makes me sway with nausea. Next best place? The hip. After much convincing, the nurse fixed the shot, swiped my skin with an alcohol pad and pushed the syringe in. The sting of a needle is never fun… but then the burning begins. It starts at the needle point with just the pinch of injection. Then, a scalding hot coin-sized circle spreads around the syringe. It rolls outward like the rings from a stone thrown into still water. Within half a minute, I feel a flaming plate pressing into my leg. Everything from the waist to the knee stings like the business end of a thousand hornets.

After just a few minutes, it is over. Yet, from the first howl that flew from my mouth, the nurse must have repeated, "I'm sorry, I'm sorry" at least 20 times.

"I'm sorry" is a phrase that is used for so many things. Think about the times you've said those words. At a funeral, "I'm sorry" means something different than it does when you accidentally bump into someone with a shopping cart, right? Sympathy and apologies are two very, very different things. A simple "I'm sorry," said once, shows compassion and helps to share your patient's pain. Say it more than once and your patient will think you did something wrong.

No one wants to be under the care of an incompetent health care professional. The more you say, "I'm sorry," the more you sound like you screwed up! Instead of apologizing, ask, "Is there anything I can do for you?" It still shows sympathy, without raising the question of fault.

CHAPTER 18

"That's What I'm Here For!"

The fluids in my stomach are sloshing like storm-tossed seas. I'm going to be sick – fast. I fumble for the nurse call button just as the shallow breaths begin. I hear her turn the corner into the room. I want to hold it in. I can't. I can't. I try, but I can't. I clamp my mouth closed, but it does no good. There's nothing I can do about it. I vomit. Hard and fast and sour.

She runs to my side. She hasn't had time to grab a pan or a tray or anything. I suck in a lungful of air filled with a chemical stench and it begins again. She makes no run for the bathroom or the supply closet. It's too late for that now. She moves to my side, wraps her hand around my forearm and lays her palm on my back. As I expel the filth from my gut, she lightly rubs my back and shoulders, paying more attention to me than the mess. I am embarrassed. I am disgusting. I am covered in putrid, chemical-filled puke. I want to cry.

Vomit is everywhere. The floor, my bed, my gown, everything.

"I'm sorry. I couldn't hold it. I tried. I'm sorry…" I mumble. I hold my dripping hands out in front of me, gesturing at the mess.

I feel, rather than hear, her cock her head with a look of surprise.

"I'm sorry, too, but only because you don't feel well. This is nothing, kiddo!" she says, still touching my back. I still want to cry. I'm ashamed. I'm gross. And now I'm so so incredibly grateful for this woman who is concerned about me, not the puddles of vomit she's standing in.

I feel so bad for giving her more to do. I apologize over and over. She stops, wipes off my chin and says, "This is nothing! Don't worry about it, okay? I just want to be sure you're all right." I give a feeble nod and drop my head to my chest.

"I'm here to take care of you. That's what I'm here for, Marcus... that's ALL I'm here for." I fight back tears.

No one wants to clean up puke, piss, shit or blood. Duh. "That isn't in my job description" is a mantra that so many hang their hats on when there's a part of the job they don't like. This nurse knows that her #1 concern is taking care of her patient. If that means a sponge bath at 3 a.m. because he puked, that's just part of it. Never a complaint, never a wrinkle of the nose, just taking care of the patient. That's your job. That's what you're there for. Help your patient by always presenting that attitude at every opportunity. Your patients will appreciate it, more than you know.

CHAPTER 19

Touch

I flinch as something brushes against my cheek.

"Sorry, Marcus," Dr. Jones, my primary plastic surgeon says. "I didn't mean to startle you."

"Ih-t's ho-kay," I rasp out through the talking trach. My words were coming easier, but the nerve damage and wired jaws still slur my speech like that of a drunkard.

"I'm going to make the incision here," he says, moving in and touching some part of my head. I can't tell exactly where because of the nerve damage, but I can feel – something – on my skull. I recoil. It's not pain, just surprise.

"Sorry, Marcus. I'll try to remember that you can't see me coming," he says. His tone isn't apologetic; more like enlightened. He's just discovered a new technique for working with this battered kid in front of him. Dr. Jones finishes the examination and turns to my parents.

"We'll need some X-rays and MRIs of Marcus' head before we do the first facial reconstruction," he says. His tone is confident and kind – exactly what a parent needs to hear before a child goes in for a 24 hour surgery.

"Where will you get the bone to fix his nose?" my father asks, worry creeping into his voice.

"Right here," Dr. Jones says, turning back to me. As he leans in, he says to me, "Touching your chest here, Marcus" A split second after he says the words, a cold, metal pen lightly glides from my armpit under my breast to my sternum. This time, I do not flinch. I'm not startled. I knew it was coming.

As a patient, one feels like they own nothing. NOTHING! Even one's own body feels like it's on loan from the hospital. Nurses, med techs, and other health care workers stroll in every day, take vitals, clean wounds, start ripping tape off of sensitive areas - and those are the violations that are the easiest to talk about! If a patient is in for anything to do with the colon or genitals, then there's an even bigger psychological risk that the patient will feel violated.

If you touch someone who does not want to be touched, that is, in most states, the crime of battery. Yet, in a hospital, a caregiver will routinely buzz into a room and automatically start pressing fingers to wrists, necks, strapping on blood pressure cuffs, all things that, if done on the street, could get the caregiver arrested.

Dr. Tim Jones also had the added complication of a patient who could not see his hands moving towards some tender area, or any area, for that matter. It took only a few flinches from the surprise of being touched until Dr. Jones began to do something that has forever secured him in my mind as the ultimate caregiver. Before he touched me in any way, he'd simply say, "Marcus, I'm going to touch your cheek, okay?" Did he always wait for a reply? No, but it gave me advanced warning that I'd soon be feeling something against my face. Plus, just by him making that statement, it showed he was taking my feelings into account.

This may be specific to me since I, of course, will never see the doctor or nurse's hands. But, I think it's a pretty good practice to keep in mind to re-spect the dignity of all patients. Touching a patient without first engaging him/her in conversation is, at best, demeaning. A few words, a quick comment about what you need to do, the simple question of, "How ya doin'?" should be enough to allow that patient to feel like they are not simply a body to be treated. And a quick, "I need to get your vitals here," a split second before strapping on a BP cuff will give a simple advanced warning about your duties at hand, which allows that patient to feel like they have some control over their own body.

CHAPTER 20

Watch Dog

It's the dead of night. I'm awake and trying to figure out the time. I know it's late because there are no visitors in my room. The floor is quiet. There's no traffic in the hallway. Insomnia has been dueling with me for weeks. Three, maybe four hours of sleep is about all I can expect, unless heavy narcotics are involved. Even then, sleep filled with hallucinations and visions isn't exactly restful.

I fumble around in the bed, my fingers spread wide to try to locate my new talking watch. The IV tubes taped to my wrists make it impossible to wear a watch like a normal person, so I just keep it in the bed. Problem is, it's just a watch – and small digital things are easily lost in the sheets and blankets. After a while, I give up. I'm awake now, I might as well ask someone. I push my right hand to the bedrail and find the nurse call button loosely wrapped around the framework. I press the button, dreading the all-too-loud speaker just a foot away from my ear.

"Yeah, Marc. Whatcha need?" shouts the voice through the speaker.

"I'm awake. I can't find my watch," I say, keeping my verbal communication as short as I can. Recently, Dr. Dennis

Fuller helped install my talking trach, but my vocal chords are still getting used to working again. After nearly a month of silence, those things had gotten lazy.

Less than a minute later, Barb walks in my room with her usual, "Hey buddy!" She walks up to my bed and says, "Can't find your watch?"

I nod.

"Okay," she says, glancing around the boom box and various medical devices on the nearby table. Seeing nothing, she starts to straighten the sheets when I hear a soft thunk of something small and flexible hitting the carpeted floor.

"There it is," I say, pointing over the edge of the bed to the floor. Barb stops. She'd heard nothing. Looking down, she finds the sought item. "Did you hear that fall or something?" she asks, bending down to retrieve the watch. I nod. "Wow. I sure didn't. It must have gotten lost in your sheet here." I nod again.

"Tell ya what, buddy, how about I fasten the watch around your friend's neck," she says, gently nudging my arm with the snout of my favorite stuffed animal. A week before, a visit from an old friend, Danielle, had been a good hour long distraction. It had also left me with a very cute stuffed animal; a bassett-looking dog with soft, floppy ears. The tag on his rump read, "Charles," but Charles is a stupid name for a dog. I hadn't thought of a name, so he'd just become, "My dog." An 18 year old guy doesn't normally need a stuffed animal for comfort, but an 18 year old guy isn't normally hooked to life support, either.

I nod at Barb as if to say, "Go ahead." She takes a few seconds, wraps the little device around the dog's spongy neck and hands it back to me. "There ya go! I know you keep your buddy with you all the time, so he'll be easier to find than just the watch, eh?" I nod again, and press the "talk" button on the watch. The digitized voice says "It's 4:42 a.m."

"Wow," I mumble to Barb, "I slept pretty long!"

Barb smiles, pleased her favorite patient has finally, finally gotten a fairly decent night's sleep.

"Need anything else?" Barb asks, giving me an affectionate tap on the knee.

"Nope, I think I've got it from here," I say, reaching towards the play button on my portable stereo.

"You know how to find me if you need anything," Barb says. She turns and exits into the hall. As soon as she's gone, I hold the dog close to my chest and press the talking button again. 4:44 a.m. I smile again. Sleep, what a concept.

Strangely enough, it wasn't the only sleep I got. A half hour of quiet Eric Clapton songs and I was snoozing again, only to be awakened by the sound of shuffling feet walking into my room.

"Marc?" my mom's quiet voice asks. "Are you asleep?"

I take a deep breath. "I was," I say, though not with the disgust I usually spew out when someone wakes me. My fingers fumble at the dog's neck. I push his silky ear to the side and press the watch's button. 6:55. "Damn!" I think, "Not bad! Not bad at all!"

My father chuckles. "Who did that for you?" he said, giving the dog a soft shake.

"Barb," I answer. "I lost my watch in the sheets. She wrapped it around his neck so I could find it. Works pretty well."

"You've got yourself a watchdog," Dad says, smiling over his own joke. I snort a short laugh. Puns are lame, but that was kinda funny. From that point on, "Charles" became known as "Watchdog." That stuffed toy brought more comfort to me on long, insomnia-filled nights than anything other than human interaction. I was never teased by my nurses or doctors, never poked fun at by my friends. Never was Watchdog anything but part of me. That's just the way it was. Watchdog was my only security blanket, my only "constant." My parents had to leave to rest, my favorite nurses worked their shifts and went home. Watchdog never left my side. Even though he wasn't sterile, surgeons allowed him in the operating room, or at least pre-op until he'd be handed (by me, of course) to my parents for safe-keeping until the recovery room. Once I was released from the hold of anesthesia, nothing gave me my feeling of wholeness again like that $10 stuffed animal.

Traumatically injured patients may grasp a security blanket of some sort. Maybe it's a stuffed animal like Watchdog, maybe it's a book they love, or maybe it's a certain shirt that makes them know they'll someday be able to wear something besides a hospital gown. Whatever their item is — respect it. Do not take it away, do not insult it, do not poke fun at it — even if it's playful teasing. That item is part of their being.

It may not be rational, it may not even make sense to you when you encounter it, but if a patient wants it nearby, provided it does not hurt their care, leave it with them. They may not verbalize this to you. Their pride may get in the way. Watch the subtle body language. Notice their vocal inflection when they ask for it. At the slightest hint of concern for an item, understand that has become their security blanket. And give it to them — it's their Watchdog.

CHAPTER 21

She Did What?

"Huh? I wonder why she did that?" the nurse asks, flipping my wrist over to inspect the IV.

"Why? What'd she do?" I ask, concerned.

"Well, usually, we'd tie off the tube on the IV, but she just taped everything over." Her tone shows bewilderment, I don't even have to see her to know her face is scrunched up with frustration. I can't give her an answer, and more than anything, I'm scared. Why? She's just told me that my previous nurse did something out of the ordinary. And all I can think about is if the IV is done improperly and falls out, I could bleed to death.

Every patient wants to feel confident they are receiving a minimum of standard care — at least! One nurse raising doubts about the actions of another ensures the patient gets the impression that the work in question was sub-par. That is a scary feeling. With their body constantly undergoing unfamiliar treatments and procedures, the patient needs to have confidence that the medical staff understands what is being done, and why. No one wants to be under the care of someone taping when they shoulda been tying.

Questioning a co-worker's job, especially when that job is dealing with the patient's body, is a big no-no. Your patient will feel as though he/she isn't getting the best care. It will also make that patient question whether or not he/she wants to be treated by the nurse in question the next time they're on duty. If there is a procedure that has been done differently, ask the patient, "Did your last nurse mention anything about your IV?" Depending on the answer, feel free to tell them that you're just making sure because you want to be certain you're informed about the situation. Plus, this is a time when you can reinforce to the patient that he/she is fine.

"Did your last nurse say anything about your IV? She taped it differently than usual and I just want to be sure there's nothing under the dressing that I could mess up. There's nothing wrong with how she did it and there's no problem. I just want to be sure there's nothing I need to be aware of before I flush the line."

This is how that interaction should have gone. It doesn't cause concern, but rather shows caring. Always ask your patient questions — they'll often have more information than you received in your report.

CHAPTER 22

Leave God Out of It

"Come on! Come on! Come on!" the nurse says, hurrying me along. Both legs are throbbing; the commode is inches, but miles, away. I breathe, heavy and fast. The sheer exertion causes sweat to trickle down my face. I'm sweating and yet, all I'm doing is moving from my bed to the commode. No human in their right mind rushes towards a commode, unless that person is busting with diarrhea. Now, this nurse is standing over me, rushing me along like a cop at an accident scene. "Nothing to see here, folks, move along, move along."

I don't like this woman. In fact, I hate her. I cannot move fast. Not because I don't want to, just because I cannot. The faster I move, the more the pain flares. Her hurrying me along results in my temper rising – fast.

"Come on, Marcus. Come on, come on!" More hurrying. My temper explodes. "Goddammit! I'm going as fast as I can! Get the hell off my back already!"

There isn't even a half second of shocked silence, but the immediate reaction of a parent who would spout out a phrase like, "You will NOT talk to me like that, young man!" There's no other way to say it – she pontificates her next words. "There's no reason for swearing, Marcus." She sounds flat, angry, personally insulted. I don't care. In fact, I'm about ready to drop a few more on her. "You don't need to use curse words, and you absolutely do not need to use the Lord's name in vain!" Now her voice is growing stronger, angrier, and more scolding. I take a deep breath, my temper reaching the boiling point.

"Look, I know I shouldn't use God's name in vain. I'm a Christian, too" I manage to get out before she cuts me off mid sentence.

"No, you're not! Not when you use language like that!" I sit down on the commode, so mad I can't speak. I am shaking with anger – literally shaking.

"Get out. Now." I jab my finger at the door. My face is fire red. If I can reach her, I will kill her.

Commodes are the most humiliating piece of equipment in a hospital, short of a proctologist's gloved index finger. Humiliation and rage and anger and loathing and hatred were stirred together in a cocktail of volatility. She knew it. And left.

No matter your faith, your religion, your idea of who "God" is or is not — never, EVER insult or question your patient's beliefs. Even if you are so so so founded in your belief, do not share your faith. No one likes to be bothered with having another's religious ideas shoved down his/her throat. That goes double for patients, who already feel vulnerable. And to insult the thoughts and opinions of something another holds so dear is the surest way to begin an adversarial relationship. And, liability. It is potentially harmful to the patient, but it's also dangerous for your job.

If the patient is religious and decides to spout his/ her beliefs, allow them to do so. Does it hurt you? No. Does it inhibit his/her healing? No. Does it annoy you? Yes... but it's your job to help promote the patient's healing. And if sharing their faith helps them to heal? Let them rant. But you, the health care worker, it is not your job to save anyone's soul. Just leave religion out of the workplace — no good can come of it.

CHAPTER 23

Who Are You?

There is a knock at my door. I turn my head to the right, almost as if I can see the doorway.

"Hi Marcus. Gene Deune, Plastic Surgery," a man's voice states. This resident has checked on me every day, but our meetings are brief and usually uninformative. He is Dr. Jones' resident and looks over Jones' work, but doesn't overstep his boundaries. He knows he is the resident and Dr. Jones is in charge. Still, he is always friendly and professional. I like him. One of the reasons is that he always identifies himself, "Gene Deune, Plastic Surgery."

Even if I were able to see him, with so many docs and nurses working on me every day, I'd do nothing more than recognize his face. But that greeting and identification, "Gene Deune, Plastic Surgery" tells me every time who I'm dealing with.

He probably does it so I know who he is. That, since I can't see, he has to repeat his name and his position. He is right. I'm still learning to identify the voices around me. I'm getting better, but with the ever-changing status of my left ear canal, sometimes it's easier than others.

If you have a long term patient, chances are, he/she is seeing multitudes of health care professionals. Every person who enters that room could easily blend together. True, sometimes a person is distinguished by their dress; a Med Tech. probably isn't wearing a white lab coat. Still, how many docs does that person see in a day, all wearing white lab coats? Reminding the traumatically injured who you are and what position you hold, as well as what you are there to do, is one way to create security in that patient's mind. Then, every time, he/she knows they are in good hands.

CHAPTER 24

"You Did Half the Work"

"**Y**ou ready to turn over, Wild Man?" Rick asks, striding up to my bedside.

"Yep, I guess so," I slur. "Let's get it over with."

This scene plays out every night; Rick helps me turn over. I've been bedridden for over a month and bedsores dot my butt like fresh acne on a teen's face. With the help of Rick, and a metal triangular shaped bar that hangs over my bed, affectionately labeled 'the jungle gym,' I roll to one side, slowly curl into the fetal position and Rick props up my back and legs with pillows. It's not perfect, but it keeps me positioned on my side – and keeps my bedsores exposed to air.

This sounds easy, right? Wrong. My newly re-built leg and face, combined with severe atrophy in the muscles, make it impossible for me to help much. My arms and chest, once able to bench press 350 lbs. now can barely lift a pillow.

Just grab onto the jungle gym when you're ready, Wild Man," Rick says, positioning himself next to me.

I reach up and find the handle. I stretch my fingers wide and wrap them tightly around the alloy bar.

"One, two, three!" Rick slowly, gently begins rotating me to my left side. At "three!" I pull down on the handle with all my might, pulling my body just a few inches off the bed. Still, through gritting teeth and a sweating forehead, Rick and I manage to expose my right hip to air, holding off the inevitable bedsores for another day.

"I don't envy you" I say, as soon as Rick "tucks me in" after the turn. "You're pushing two bills over there, stud," I say, making a joke of just how macho Rick is, while at the same time silently crying how my own muscles have melted away.

"Nah, you did half the work, Wild Man," he said, giving my shoulder a playful punch.

In weeks, I'd gone from an all-American teenage guy who looked like he should be on a football field, to an invalid. Invalid. In valid. That's what my life felt like. No one was more horrified at a pre-maturely aged body than yours truly. No one, especially me, wanted to think I had no muscles left to even lift myself. Yet, it was true — and Rick knew it. His "white lie" helped secure my self-image; an idea that I still had some part of my old self left.

One might say Rick was lying to me and that lying is never, EVER an option. A lie isn't a lie when everyone knows it's not the truth. Rick knew it, I knew it, everyone knew it. But Rick wouldn't allow me to think I was much less than the man I'd been weeks before. Even if we all knew the truth, Rick wouldn't bring it into the open. There was no need. We just played our roles; he as the helper, me as the person in control of my body.

CHAPTER 25

Patients Don't Make Medical Ethics Calls

"There's a kid downstairs, Marcus," the nurse says, taping an IV to my arm. "Everyone in his family are Christian Scientists and their religion won't let them receive blood. This poor kid is going to die if he doesn't get the blood, and there's nothing anyone can do about it." She finishes taping me up and waits for my response. I simply nod. I have no opinion. I don't want to tell her what is right and what is wrong for someone else. I don't want to think about another kid dying who might be the same as me. I don't want to know if he does, in fact, drop dead. I just don't want to know.

That's not to say I don't care. I do. Too much, probably. But I can't spend energy being concerned about this other kid when I'm struggling myself. I need to feel like my caregiver is not worrying about someone else, but is focusing her attention on me. Not a dying kid, not her next coffee break, me. Just me.

This nurse's heart was in the right place. I can see the little gerbil wheel in her brain turning and saying, "I'll tell Marcus about this other kid, then he'll want to get better." Maybe, maybe not. First of all, I'm so close to death that the idea of actually thinking about another kid is more than I can bare. Second, the debate of medical ethics should be done by doctors and philosophers and lawyers and the people involved – not by patients confined to hospital beds.

However, the most important bit of this interaction is this: telling me about other patients means that, even when you're with me, you're not with me. I need your care to be concentrated on me, Marcus, not elsewhere. Plus, if she's telling me about him, what's to say she's not telling him about me? I don't want to think about her saying, "Hey little Christian Scientist kid, I've got a patient upstairs who is blind because someone got drunk and hit him..." Please!

Your patient does not need to make medical ethics calls for anyone but him/herself. To ask them to even comment on such a debate is asking that patient to put his/her own needs on a backburner during such a critical time. Commenting on someone who isn't immediately involved with his/her care is unproductive. Not that the other person's life has no meaning, but the severely injured patient needs to worry about nothing but his/her own healing.

CHAPTER 26

Tell Me, for God's Sake!

I wait. And I wait. And I wait some more. I am in pain. Every square inch of my body is filled with a hammering sensation that is the result of yet another hefty surgery. Only this time, the surgeons saw fit to release me from the O.R. after 12 hours, not 15 plus like the last few times.

"I need pain meds," I'd said to the nurse. She promised to get them. Here I sit. No medicine, now some 45 minutes later. With every second that passes, I hurt more. And more. And more. I want to kill her for making me wait, for making me suffer. But, I cannot kill she who is not here.

Thirty minutes later, she arrives. I'm so angry, so frustrated, so seething with hatred for this suffering that I cannot even form words. If she gets one step closer to the bed, I'll not be able to control my hands. I'm scared. I'm scared that I will reach out, grab her by the neck and choke her. I would, that is, if it didn't hurt so much to move.

"I'm sorry I took so long, Marcus," she says, popping the plastic cap off of a syringe. She says nothing more for a few seconds as she concentrates on injecting the gift into my I.V.

"I looked to see what meds were ordered for you and, well, there was nothing. How many surgeons worked on you today? Four or five?" she asked, turning her attention to me and finishing her job. I nod and shrug. How the hell should I know? I was asleep.

"Yeah, I guess they got their wires crossed and no one actually submitted orders. So, I had to call your main surgeon and tell him the situation. He wrote the orders, but it just takes some time to get those up, to get the meds documented, all that stuff. I knew you were in a lot of pain, so I tried to get it done as quickly as I could. Sorry that took so long, kiddo," she says, patting me on the arm.

Mere moments before, I'd wanted her dead, cold corpse stomped into the ground. The frustration and angst was nearly as bad as the pain. And why was I mad? Misperception. She'd been on my side all along, doing the legwork to correct someone else's mistake... but I didn't know that. To pop into my room and say, "I haven't forgotten about you. I just had to get an order for your meds," would have left me frustrated, but not at the wrong person. I felt as though I'd been kept in the dark, forgotten, disregarded.

Never leave your patient twisting in the wind. If a task is going to take longer than thought, simply tell him or her that "I'm on it, it's just going to take a few more minutes than I expected." The comfort that you are not forgotten makes things more bearable.

CHAPTER 27

Thunk

Thunk! I hear a muffled sound just inches from my face. I stop. "What was that?" I ask, "My face??"

Rick glances up and sees the triangular bar swinging from its chain just inches from my head. I hear him chuckle. The situation can't be too dire.

"Yep, Wild Man, it sure was! Stick your hand out and see what you hit," he says. He is amused. I'm too afraid to laugh yet, but the fear is starting to slip away with each of Rick's laughs. Cautiously, I extend my fingers.

I find a cold, metal handle-still swinging from the jungle gym. I grasp the heavy duty alloy bar and stop its movement.

Man this thing could really do some damage! I press my fingers to my forehead, checking for blood. Finding none, and unable to even feel the impact due to neuropathy, I decide to make light of it.

"Thank God for nerve damage! It's a good thing I can't feel that or I'd be screaming to wake the dead!" Just a week ago, I'd have thrown a tantrum of childlike proportions. Now, my amusement shows Rick his patient is progressing – and fast.

"Yeah, and if you were deaf, you wouldn't have even heard that *thunk* at all!" Rick says, giving me a light punch on the shoulder.

Through the rest of the turning ritual, Rick and I talk, joke, laugh and do everything we can to make the hour-long task easier. This happens several times each night. I am really, really sick of having to expose my bedsore-riddled butt to another man. Still, better Rick than some hottie little nursie-pooh. Sometimes, when our competition of wit is heated, I can almost forget I am blind... almost.

"You going to try to get some sleep, Wild Man?" Rick asks. He gave me this nickname the first night I was under his care. He hasn't forgotten. I haven't either. I doubt I ever will. The war with insomnia still gives battle; my nights and days are completely screwed up.

"Chances are, I'll be awake all damned night once again," I say, frustration already setting in.

"Give me a little while to get some stuff taken care of. I'll stop in a little later and see if you're still awake. If you are, I'll hang out for a while," Rick says. It is like music to my ears!

For the next hour, I try to fall asleep. Relaxation exercises, self-hypnosis, counting sheep, nothing works. I give up. As if on schedule, an hour later, Rick walks in.

"Still not asleep, Wild Man?" There is sympathy in his voice.

"Nope!" I respond with more than a hint of exasperation." Think you could punch me really hard and knock me out?" I ask, only half joking.

"I think Dr. Jones would have me by the balls if I ruined his work on your face!" Rick says, chuckling and pulling up a chair.

For the next hour, Rick and I talk about growing up. We share similar stories of our teenage years of parties, girls, more parties, and more girls. We talk of the nursing profession, his choice to leave the corporate world behind and become a nurse, as well as a bit of gossip about his co-workers.

Although Rick was close to 20 years my senior, he treated me as he would any other adult. During these conversations my blindness slowly became irrelevant. Rick and I were just two friends, swapping tales as if one of us wasn't disabled or injured at all. Those things that had governed my life over the past month were now simply non-issues. Those 60 minutes of conversation were more precious than any tangible gift I could receive.

As in every job, health care will have times when you're busier than a one-legged man in an ass kicking contest, and other times where you're wishing for some excitement. The more time you can spend with your patient, the more they feel cared for. Provided that patient isn't trying to sleep or visit with others, when you can, spend a little extra time with him/her. You may never know just how much those few extra moments of attention mean to your patients.

CHAPTER 28

"This Might Work Better"

I move my hands forward onto the padded grips of the walker. Walker. Wretched piece of metal. Eighteen year old guys should NOT be seen using one of these things; these horrible instruments of the old. I suck in a lungful of antiseptic-laden air and try to push my 200 plus pound body off of the bed. The walker rocks backward, precarious like a boulder on the edge of a mountain.

"Here," the physical therapist says, "This might work better." With that, she moved the metal frame closer to the bed, encasing me in the skeleton of a metal coffin. "I'll hold my hand right here," she says, tapping the top bar mid-way between the grips. "Lots of times, it helps to get it as close to you as you can, then press directly down. The closer you get it to you, the easier it'll be to go straight up. Want to give it a try?" I nod and slowly, deliberately suck in another lungful of oxygen. With far less effort, I begin to rise into place. I smile. I actually smile.

"Good job!" she says, still holding onto the walker.

When a patient tries unsuccessfully to perform some sort of action, suggest — rather than cor-

rect. The physical therapist gave me a tip and I, of course, chose to implement that idea. However, would I have been so ready to try if she'd have said, "It's not working because the walker is too far away"? No. In fact, the average patient would not take this as a statement of the obvious, but rather criticism. Here, she made a suggestion that, as she explained, often helps others. This shows it's a tried and true manner that patients just like me have found successful. It will always, always motivate your patients when they feel empowered to choose.

CHAPTER 29

Parting Shots

The alcohol pad is cold and wet and clean. The nurse says nothing, just continues to swipe the cotton pad back and forth over my hand. I.V. time. Again. The I.V. antibiotics are so strong that, after 24 hours, the vein in which the I.V. was inserted will collapse. Then, it's I.V. time again. And it hurts. Horribly.

All right, you're going to feel a little bee sting on the back of your hand, Marcus," she says.

Yeah, right, I think. The I.V. "bee stings" term has long since lost its effectiveness. Now, it's just pain and pain and more pain.

The nurse says, "Okay, we'll do it on three." I take a deep breath. She begins to count. Slowly, carefully, "One." Slight pause. I begin to feel the hot fluid press into my skin. "Two," she relays. The sting grows hotter. I grit my teeth together. "Three," she says. I squeeze my opposite hand into a fist as she says three. In less than one second after saying, "three," the nurse smiles and says, "All done!" There is still a bit of a burning in the back of my hand, but the worst is over. And it wasn't so bad.

She chatters away and tapes the tubes to my forearms. "That wasn't so bad, was it, Marcus?" she asks.

"No, not at all!" I smile. I'm humbled. I feel as though I was making a mountain out of a molehill. It DID hurt, but certainly not as bad as the others. Why? As the nurse finished her work, I sat thinking over the exchange. Two days ago when this same thing happened, I was screaming to wake the dead. Was it because this one is in the back of my hand, and the other was under my wrist? Maybe, but that hardly seems likely. Maybe it was the nurse herself. Or maybe it's a different medicine. I couldn't figure it out.

Then, I slow my mental rewind. When she said "one," I was already starting to feel the pressure in my hand. I thought it was only her thumb pressed into my skin, but the more I think about it, the more I'm convinced that's not right. In fact, I'm pretty sure she stuck me as soon as she said, "One." I feel a little duped, but it's duped to control my pain. By the time she'd said "two," it was as good as over. I grinned, ready to congratulate her on her slyness.

The few moments a patient has leading up to the shot are filled with apprehension and tension. Yet, like with most things, the thing we fear often turns out to be overshadowed by the fear itself. Then, when the event finally happens, relief is immediate. And we're grateful that our fears were mostly unfounded.

Your patient will be filled with apprehension when he/she knows a needle of any type is coming. Even if they've gotten used to it, there is still that split second wonder, "Will it hurt worse this time?" You can control this situation by giving your patient a countdown... and then do the deed before they know what's going on. A pleasant surprise is always welcome.

CHAPTER 30

When a Cigar Is
Just a Cigar

"Well, Marcus, how've you been lately?" asks the even, gentle voice.

"I'hum betta," I say, still working at forming words with a re-built face and nerve damage.

"The last time I was in here, you were still writing and talking about killing yourself," he prods.

"I got betta," I say, mocking an English accent and landing a line from a Monty Python movie. He doesn't get it. Oh well, win some, lose some.

"You know, your improvement is nothing short of dramatic," he says happily. "When I first saw you, you were on oxygen, you couldn't talk, your ear just looked like a piece of hamburger hanging off your head. Now, look at you!" I decide not to share the obvious – if I could look at myself, I wouldn't be here now.

"Thanks," I mutter, not knowing what to say.

Dr. McCoy, a psychiatrist, has been in here before. It's been a while, but a single day feels like a million years in my world. Barb told me a few nights ago that she thinks I'll soon be getting out of here. Maybe McCoy does, too, and this is an exit interview, of sorts; just to be sure I don't go home and blow my fool head off or something.

"And who's this fellow next to you?" Dr. McCoy asks, nuzzling Watchdog's floppy ears over my wrist.

"This is Watchdog," I say, pulling my favorite security blanket closer to me.

"Oh, is that because since you can't see, he watches out for you?" Dr. McCoy asks, genuinely thinking he's hit on something sub-conscious.

"No" I snort a laugh. "It's because he has a watch around his neck!" As I'm saying it in the most mocking tone I can find, Dr. McCoy realizes his mistake. I make fun of him with my tone, but that's the extent of where I'll take it. His heart is in the right place, but sorry, Doc, sometimes a cigar is just a cigar!

Even if you are a trained psychotherapist, don't assume you can easily get inside your patient's head. When I first met Dr. McCoy, it was soon after I began scrawling, "I want to die, I want to die!" on my tablet. The staff immediately sent him to my bedside to keep me from doing anything dire. Even in the horrible state I was just a week post-crash, I knew I couldn't kill myself. I couldn't lift my head off of a pillow, much less run to the window, open it and fling myself down seven stories to the street. As with most psychotherapists, Dr. McCoy showed himself to be a great listener. This was one example where his mouth ran faster than his mind. If he'd have taken an extra second to glance at Watchdog, he'd have seen a large, plastic watch wrapped around the dog's neck. Since he did not, it left me feeling all the more like I was being analyzed.

Don't assume your patient has problems that are obvious to you. If a burn victim with fresh scars is on your floor, you may assume those wounds are the reason he/she is there. Until you see that he/she is in a fresh leg cast. The old saying, "To assume makes an ass out of you and me" applies as well in medical settings, as it does in the outside world.

CHAPTER 31

Birds of a Feather

"I tried to get in here earlier to drop off some mail, but there were so many people around that I couldn't even get to your bed!" the nurse says brightly, depositing the envelopes onto the bedside table. "Who were all those guys?"

"Buddies from high school," I say, smiling a bit at the memory from just a few hours earlier. The nurse giggles.

"There were so many guys in here, it was like walking into a frat house or something!" "Yeah, kinda," I mutter, all of my energy drained from the visit and onslaught of friends.

"And you know what? Every one of those guys came up and thanked me for helping you," she says, still smiling. "I've never seen a group of young men that are that polite. You really, really have some special people around you, Marcus!"

I nodded. I knew all too well that my friends and family were having to step up to the plate. One of their own was down and it was the best they could do to try to pick him back up. But, it didn't feel like obligation. Every person who stepped through the threshold of my hospital room was there because they loved me. And I them. You can't drag a person into a friendship. I was so focused on my own healing that it wasn't for many, many years that I fully understood the sacrifices they all made. And, to this day, I am humbled by their actions.

At the time, though, for others to compliment my friends and visitors did one thing: it complimented me. Especially with young patients, there's a "team" mentality – all for one and one for all, compliment us and it compliments me, insult me and it insults us, that sort of thing. In essence, this nurse was telling me that I, too, was a polite, courteous young man – a cut above the rest of guys our age.

I'm certainly not suggesting you go above and beyond the realms of good taste. No one would expect you to lie about those gathered around your patient. Still, finding some way to compliment the visitors, but say the compliment to the patient, is key. Even if it's nothing more than, "It's so great to see you have so much support!"

If you can compliment how nice the visitors are, even better. Even comments on their physical appearance help young patients to feel like they're one with the in crowd. I knew that one of my nurses was on my side when she said, "Was the brunette in here earlier your sister? She's really pretty!"

Why does this matter? It shows you're taking an interest in your patient's life — not just his/her care. It helps reinforce that you know that outside the hospital, your patient is a person; a person with friends, family and connections. Again, respecting the patient as a person, not just a body to be cared for, is a key element in helping that person recover.

CHAPTER 32

Work Me In

It's been two weeks since I was discharged from the hospital. Two weeks that I've sat in my parents' living room and, for the first time in two months, been allowed to sleep through the night. I'm excited about being home, but it's also still busy. I may not be "in" Barnes Hospital any more, but I'm still there two or three times per week. Like I am today.

This morning, my family made the hour long drive to Barnes once again. I'm seeing Dr. Jones and we'll schedule my next facial surgery. After that, I have a three hour break until I see the oral surgeon. Then, an hour later, I'll be headed up to the ENT floor to see Dr. Neely, the doc who calls me "senor." It is going to be a long, long day.

As we're walking through the hospital, I hear a booming voice barreling down the hallway, "Hey Marc dude! What's up, man?" It is, of course, Dennis Fuller. My talking trach is still in place and my words are more enunciated every day. We shake hands and catch up. I haven't seen him since the day before I left the hospital. I explain that I have three doctor appointments over the next six hours. I need the healing, but no one, NO ONE wants to sit around a hospital for six hours.

"This is ridiculous," Dennis says, turning and gesturing for us to follow. "Let's see if we can shorten your stay."

He leads us into an office and right up to the secretary's desk. "Can you get me ENT on the phone?" The secretary knows Dennis and happily complies, pressing a button and handing the phone to the big man.

"Hi Julie," he says to the secretary. "Dr. Neely has an appointment with Marcus Engel today. These folks have a long drive and a bunch of other appointments today. Can you work him in earlier?" Thirty seconds later, he turns to me and proclaims, "Neely in half an hour!" before I can thank him he turns back to the secretary. "Now, how about Dr. Beehner in oral surgery." It's a command more than a request, but an order the secretary is happy to fill. Why? Because he's Dennis and he wants to help. Again, she hits some buttons and hands him the phone.

"This is Dr. Fuller with speech path. Marcus Engel has an appointment later. Can you get him in any earlier? This kid just got out of the hospital and he needs to be home more than he needs to be here." I am almost crying with happiness when he turns to me again, "Beehner as soon as you're done with Neely. Dennis has just taken a six hour day of waiting and worrying down to a 90 min. slot with three different docs. Is he able to do this because he's a doc making the request of other docs? Maybe, but maybe not.

If a patient says they will already be at the hospital and they want an appointment to fit their schedule, please, please try to make that appointment. In our case, it was a combination of reasons that made this so special: I was still hurt, I had to see many doctors, I couldn't walk and I had to inconvenience both parents to have my own appointment. While this isn't the standard with most patients, if they request a certain time slot, do your best to fulfill it. Your job is to gather information and see how desperately that person needs that time slot. Do not simply look at a schedule and say, "The doctor is booked solid that day." The patient's mental health is so quickly aided by the shortened "day of doctors" experience.

CHAPTER 33

Don't Hold Grudges

"**M**arcus, I can't tell you how much your attitude has improved since I started seeing you," Dr. Gay says, positioning my chair and the light overhead.

"You've gotten better, yourself," I say. We both laugh a little.

"Yeah, I was pretty rough on you the first couple of times you were in here," he says, leaning down over my chair. I tilt my head back and open my jaw, but not before I shrug a little. All is forgiven – nearly a year later, all is forgiven.

The first time I'd been rolled into Dr. Gay's office, I wasn't happy. Not even close. I knew dental impressions were coming. And anything to do with the tender, nerve damaged area below my nose and above my chin was off limits for everyone. Even myself. I hated touching that part of my face and not being able to feel my fingertips on my cheek. I hated the odd sensation of the nerves being excited artificially, usually by electrodes stuck to every square inch of skin from the chin on up. And I really, really hated the idea of someone poking their fingers around in my mouth when the nerves AND the chipped fragments of teeth joined forces to make it the most uncomfortable part of an already aching face.

When he'd entered, Dr. Gay had introduced himself, pulled up a chair and told me to open my mouth. A command, not a request. I obeyed, but not happily. The next thing I knew, there was a plastic tray shoved into my pallet. The hard plastic edges scraped the tender skin grafted area to the roof of my mouth. The impression goo seeped down the back of my throat. I was taken completely off guard by this wretched experience and, as I screamed through my nose, Dr. Gay shoved a finger in my mouth and pressed the impression tray back into its intended position. I thrashed and jerked; not going so far as to hit him, but he could tell I wanted to throw punches. And I would have – except that Dr. Gay was my last hope of being able to eat solid food once again. His specialty as a maxillofacial prosthodontist rendered him such a hot commodity that there was no one else to turn to. And, if I lipped off much more to him, I'd run the chance of him refusing to treat me. *Screw it*, I thought, *he's getting a piece of my mind anyway*. Then, the barrage of curses began.

"There's to be no cussing in this office," he said, sounding like he was lecturing a child. *You let someone shove a bunch of crap down your throat and we'll see if you get pissed*, I thought. I said nothing, though, trying to be adult about it. It was NOT the beginning of a beautiful friendship.

Now, a year later, I'm back. I've sat in this chair no less than a dozen times since that initial meeting. Gradually, Dr. Gay and I have come to an understanding. We're not best buds, but we respect each other. He now moves slowly and takes time to explain what he's about to do. And, if I flinch from pain, he apologizes, usually with some comment like, "I know this isn't comfortable…"

In the last year, Dr. Gay has taken a mangled mess of a mouth and provided me with the ability to, once again, eat solid food. It's going to take some getting used to, but the idea I'll be able to eat something that hasn't been turned to mush pleases me beyond belief.

"Yeah, you are like a whole different person," he says, grabbing some instruments from the dental tray.

At the end of the appointment, he stands and shakes my hand. "I'll need to see you when you're back at Christmas, okay?" I nod and shake his hand. "Take care of yourself out there… and try to have a little fun while you're at it."

He has just signed my walking papers. I am now considered medically healed enough to start the process of returning to college. I can eat solid food once again – that which has been holding me hostage for the last 12 months. I smile as I walk out of his office.

It's unrealistic to think all human interactions will get off on the right foot. Mine sure didn't with Dr. Gay. In fact, for a time, there was no one in the world I hated more than him. Yes, those were the messed up thoughts of an injured kid, but it didn't seem irrational to me. Even with my deplorable behavior, Dr. Gay didn't hold a grudge. Maybe it was because we both realized we should have done things differently upon our first meeting, but either way, by the end of the process, we became as close to friends as one can get with their physician.

When you work with patients, even if the first interaction isn't positive, treat the next like it is the first. Sooner or later, there'll be some sort of break in the defenses of the patient. And when there is, you'll stand tall, knowing you helped their healing process.

Epilogue

So, there you have it; a long, traumatic hospitalization experience from the perspective of a critically ill patient – me. Am I so different from the many patients you treat? Sure, in some ways. But in many ways we, the patients, are all the same: all dependant on you for our quality of life, and often, our very survival.

My hope is that you can walk away from this book with at least one new idea to implement in your duties as a health-care professional. Not only to help your patients, but I want to help you, too. And why do I care about you? Easy – you are the incarnation of these characters. You are: Dr. Jones, Barb, Rick, Betty, Rita and many, many more all rolled up into one. You may not see yourself that way, but I, as a patient, do. I, and all other patients, look to their caregivers as more than just those who take vitals and pass out pills. We look to you for compassion, for assistance, for reassurance and for hope. We look to you to hold our hand when we're afraid, to be the punching bag that absorbs our necessary outbursts, and as a friendly shoulder, there for us. Unless you've lived at the other end of the stethoscope, you may not fully comprehend all the roles you fill. Hopefully, this book gives you a bit of the patient's perspective.

Now, because you are all caregivers rolled into one… I thank you. Yes, you. You the person holding this book. You, the one who looked at a specific story from this book and thought, "Ya know, I'm going to give that a try!" You, the person who takes care of people like me. You have a tough, tough job. You've chosen a field with many headaches and potentially few rewards. I hope this book is, in some way, a reward to you. An acknowledgement for doing what you do, helping those during the most difficult times and caring with compassion and thoughtfulness – even when it is not easy. Thank you for what you do.

Thank you, thank you and thank you.

www.MarcusEngel.com

&

www.MarcusEngel.Blogspot.com

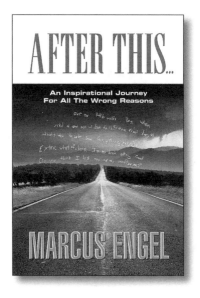